Better Home

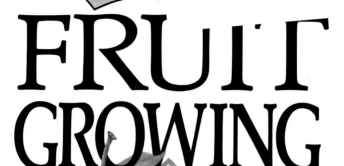

FRUIT GROWING

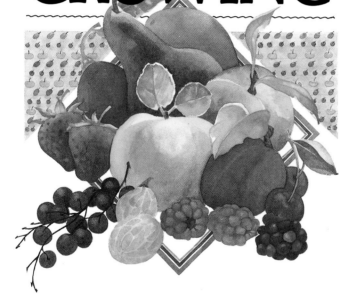

MURDOCH BOOKS
Sydney • London

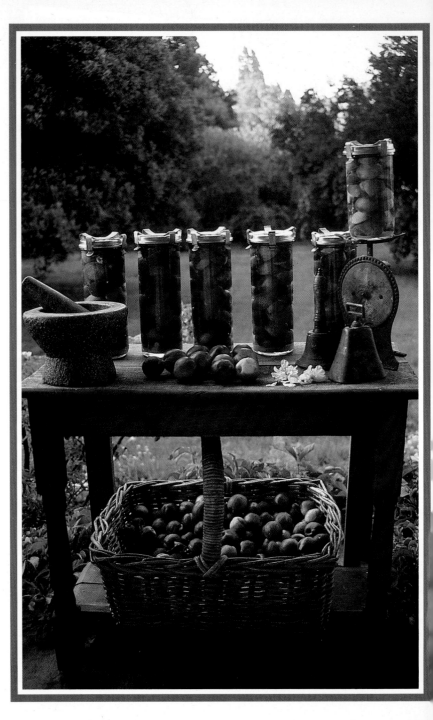

Contents

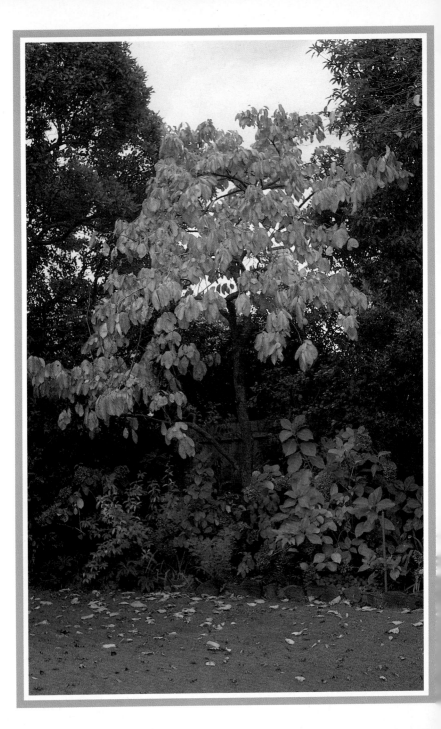

FRUIT
producing your own

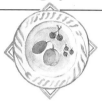

I t can be very rewarding to grow your own fruit, whether it be a humble lemon to flavour seafood, a crispy apple for a school lunch or a few nutritious avocados to serve as a first course at dinner.

Fruit trees are beautiful — some have decorative, glossy foliage or brilliant autumn-toned leaves, others provide showy spring blossom, while the citrus group is eye-catching all year round. Some are so spectacular in fruit that they make excellent specimen plants in lawns or courtyards.

Fruit trees can be grown in most areas of Australia. They are not difficult to cultivate but it pays to do a little research as to what varieties produce top quality fruit in your locality. Temperature, frost and rainfall are basic considerations in selecting the right kind of fruit trees for your area.

Space is often limited in home gardens and it may be difficult to find accommodation, as fruit trees should never be over-crowded. Consider carefully the ultimate height and spread of each one. If your backyard is already overcrowded, try the front garden and grow only one or two of your favourites as specimen fruit trees.

Some fruit trees may be grown in containers with good results, as long as varieties are carefully chosen. Their aesthetic appeal — attractive shape, fragrant flowers and spectacular display — can be used to advantage on a terrace or in a sheltered courtyard.

When choosing fruit trees, the most important point is that you plant varieties you and your family prefer to eat.

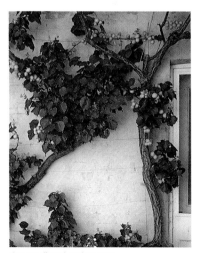

An espaliered apricot tree.

CITRUS TREES
ornamental evergreens

The citrus family is one of the easiest groups to grow and is most often cultivated in the home garden. Citrus trees are ornamental, highly productive and have delightfully fragrant blossoms. All citrus are evergreen and vary from medium-sized, shapely trees to small compact shrubs, some of which make ideal container specimens. Rich in vitamin C, many citrus fruits can be picked progressively over a lengthy period. They usually begin fruiting within two or three years of planting.

Climate, Position and Soil

Citrus fruit will do well in temperate to warm climates and prefer relatively frost-free areas with short winters. They are excellent for coastal zones but will grow inland where winters are mild and plenty of water is available. They grow less well in cold mountainous districts, where severe frosts may damage the trees and fruit.

All citrus do best in an open, sunny position with good drainage and protection from strong winds. They are surface-rooting and prefer light, sandy loam soils. If soil is heavy, dig in plenty of organic matter mixed with sand. If a citrus tree is grown as a lawn specimen ensure that grass is kept at least 40 cm away from the young trunk until the tree is well-established.

Planting

Do not allow the roots of trees to dry out on the way home from the nursery or before you have a chance to plant them. An early spring planting is best when the risk of frost has passed but before the weather becomes too warm.

Remove the tree from the container and gently tease out any pot-bound roots. Dig a hole wide enough to spread out the roots comfortably to the same depth as they were in the container. Be careful not to cover the budded graft union when filling in the hole with soil. Gradually fill the hole with compost-enriched soil, treading it down firmly. Water well. After planting, spread mulch around the base of the tree but keep it well away from the trunk to avoid collar rot. Do not feed until the plant is thoroughly established.

Management

All citrus need a year-round supply of water. Give a good soaking during dry weather and maintain mulch around young trees as an ideal way to conserve moisture.

Apply fertiliser one year after planting. Ready-mixed citrus fertilisers are available from nurseries. Apply as directed in early spring and again in early autumn. The feeding roots of citrus are located around the tree under the outer foliage canopy. Always make sure that the soil is watered well both before and after applying fertiliser.

Citrus trees do not need regular pruning and are only pruned when necessary. If growth is overcrowded, thin inside twigs and limbs to allow a free passage of air and sunlight. Remove any shoots and suckers from a low position on the stem and make sure that all broken limbs and dead wood are removed.

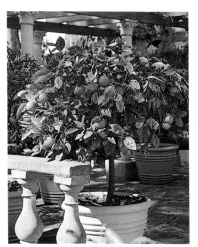

Citrus trees such as this tangelo thrive in pots and look extremely decorative.

Citrus Trees in Containers

Pots and tubs can be used for growing some kinds of citrus. They are ideal for the small city garden. Choose varieties carefully ensuring that they are adaptable to pots. The container needs to be a generous size. Soil must be well-drained with a good moisture-retaining material such as peatmoss or well-rotted compost. Soil moisture quickly becomes depleted in pots and in hot dry weather a daily watering might be necessary. Container-grown citrus need small amounts of fertiliser frequently. Slow-release fertilisers are particularly good as they provide nutrients continuously for a number of months. Always water before scattering the fertiliser, fork it in and water deeply again. Suitable citrus trees for containers include Meyer lemon, Tahiti lime, kumquats, tangelo and mandarin.

Controlling Diseases and Pests

Many people prefer not to use chemicals in their gardens at all. Chemicals are dangerous and should be labelled correctly and stored out of the reach of children. By law, however, you must spray fruit fly and codling moth. When using chemicals, it is essential to thoroughly spray the tree with pesticide from top to bottom. Make sure that the right materials are used at the right rate at the right time and that the job is done thoroughly. Products are available in home garden pack sizes. Specific chemicals are not recommended in this book as applications and application rates vary from State to State. Write to your State department of agriculture or see your local nursery to check what is currently recommended for a particular fruit for your area. State pesticide registers are updated from time to time, as more information and new, more effective products become available.

Black Spot and Melanose: Small brown or black spots appear on fruit, and leaves may wilt. Remove leaves and spray fruit with a fungicide.

Citrus Scab: Scabby or warty growth appears on tree and fruit. Treat with an appropriate spray.

Rots: Collar rot, stem rot and root rot are caused by the fungus *Phytophthora* which attacks the conducting tissues of the plant, causing it to decline and often completely collapse. Ensure that the bud union is well clear of the ground and that the tree never becomes waterlogged. Treat affected areas by cutting away dead bark to expose healthy wood beneath. Coat with a recommended fungicide.

Many insects have natural predators such as birds. With fruit trees, however, birds, may be *another* pest with which you have to contend. Many home gardeners grow their fruit under nets. While citrus trees are not especially attractive to birds, which seem to prefer much softer skinned pome and berry fruits, if you are grouping your fruit trees together in a small orchard under a net, you may have to contend with the following pests:

Black Citrus Aphids: These can attack the young growing shoots in autumn. Blast them off with a hose or spray with insecticide.

Fruit Fly: A serious pest which attacks many kinds of fruit. The wasp-like fly lays eggs in the developing fruit. Spray with the insecticide recommended in your State and observe the withholding period. All infected fruit, whether on the tree or on the ground, should be destroyed by burning or boiling. The New South Wales department of agriculture suggests a good clean method of destruction is to secure the fruit inside a sealed plastic bag and expose it to the sun long enough to kill the larvae.

Mealy Bugs: These tiny white insects are surrounded by a waxy substance. Spray with insecticide.

Scale: Insects such as citrus red scale, white wax, black and white louse can be controlled by thoroughly drenching the tree with an appropriate spray.

Spined Citrus Bug and Bronze Orange Bug: When mature, these attack citrus trees causing wilting of the young shoots and flower stalks. Hose off with water or use a recommended treatment.

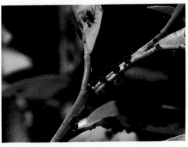

Aphids can be hosed off.

Grapefruit

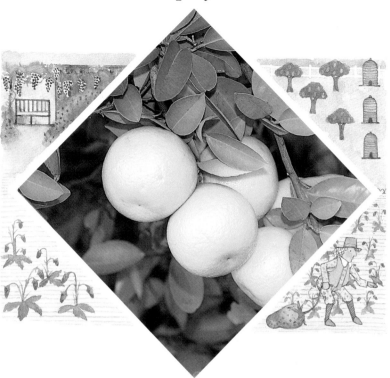

Grapefruit (*Citrus paradisi*) is an attractive evergreen tree growing 5–12 m with fragrant white blossom in spring. Thrives in tropical and sub-tropical areas; frost-tender.

Origin: East Asia or, according to some authorities, the West Indies.

Varieties: Marsh Seedless — very popular, fruiting late summer to autumn; Wheeny — good for cooler climates, late spring to early autumn; New Zealand — orange-coloured flesh with excellent juice, mid-spring to midsummer; Thompson — good for inland areas. Most varieties fruit only at the end of the second year.

Planting: Plant in full sun, in deep, well-drained soil.

Cultivation: Keep well-watered, especially during hot weather. Mulch to destroy weeds and avoid damaging surface roots. Fertilise in spring and autumn with citrus food. Protect from fruit fly in coastal areas.

Harvesting: Leave fruit on the tree until ripe and well-coloured. Fruit can be frozen if peeled and cut into segments. Grapefruit is extremely popular as a breakfast fruit, its slightly acidic flavour providing an invigorating start to the day. Alternatively, it makes a refreshing entrée.

Kumquat

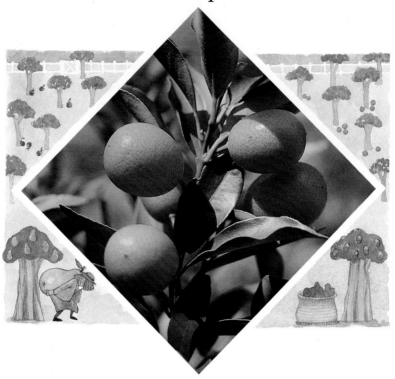

Kumquats (*Fortunella* species) make delightful, compact, evergreen container or small garden specimens to 2 m. They have clusters of scented white flowers in spring and summer and grow in most climates being very adaptable trees.

Origin: China, Japan, Malaysia.

Varieties: Meiwa — good for cold, frosty areas, flowers profusely in summer, rounded fruit in early spring to mid-autumn; Marumi — round fruits, early spring to mid-autumn; Nagami — bright orange, oval fruit which matures over a long period.

Planting: Plant in well-composted soil. If growing in pots, make sure you provide plenty of good quality soil mixed with sand and compost or well-rotted manure. Plant firmly.

Cultivation: Keep well-watered in hot weather. Mulch and feed in spring and autumn with citrus food.

Harvesting: Pick fruit when ripe and well-coloured, as needed. Kumquats make an excellent marmalade and delicious homemade kumquat brandy. Kumquats also make good presents as highly attractive bottled preserved fruit in glass jars at Christmas time, for birthdays or on other special occasions.

Lemon

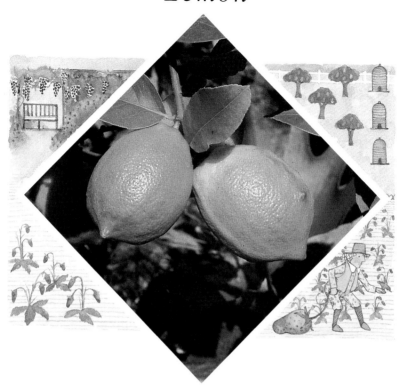

E very garden large or small should have room for a lemon tree (*Citrus limon*). Lemon trees reach about 6 m high and can be grown in all climates, depending on variety.

Origin: Uncertain, possibly India or perhaps China.

Varieties: Eureka — a vigorous grower, crops all year round, good for coastal districts; Lisbon — a thorny variety, tolerates light frosts and crops in autumn; Meyer — an adaptable hybrid more tolerant of climate extremes, crops in summer and is a good container plant.

Planting: Plant in full sun, in well-composted soil which does not need to be very deep, one of the reasons lemons grow well in large pots.

Cultivation: Water well in hot weather. Mulch to conserve water and smother weeds. Feed in spring and autumn with citrus food. Protect from citrus scab.

Harvesting: Leave fruit on tree until ripe and pick as need arises. Store in an airy spot free of draughts. Lemons can be used to make pomanders — stuck with cloves, rolled in orris root powder (available from health food stores) and placed in drawers or wardrobes to scent your clothes.

Lime

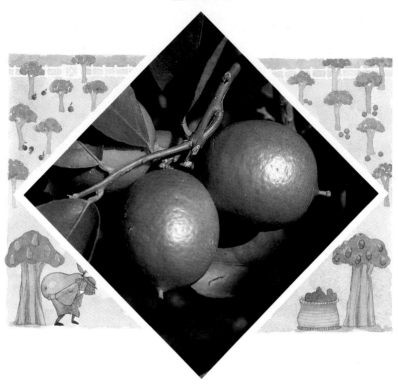

Attractive limes (*Citrus auranti-folia*) grow about 3–4 m high and have fragrant white blossom throughout the year. Limes are frost-sensitive and do best in tropical and warm coastal regions.

Origin: Tropical areas of Asia.

Varieties: Tahiti — seedless, almost thornless, good container crop, fruits mostly in winter but may crop all year in some areas; West Indian lime — small, acidic fruit not recommended for home gardens as it is susceptible to tristeza virus infection; Rangpur — mandarin-lime hybrid, suitable for using in drinks. Kusai lime — lime-kumquat hybrid, suitable for using in marmalades and preserves.

Planting: Plant in full sun, in well-composted soil. Limes make excellent, long-lived tub specimens for courtyards, sunny balconies or in small inner city gardens.

Cultivation: Keep well-watered; mulch and feed in spring and autumn with citrus food. Protect from aphids.

Harvesting: Limes drop their fruit quickly when mature so ideally fruit should be harvested when slightly under-ripe. Limes can be used to 'cook' raw fish, and in drinks, jams, pies and other desserts.

Mandarin

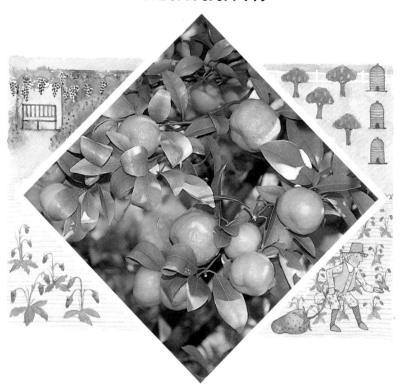

M andarins (*Citrus reticulata*) have a wider climatic range than oranges. Small evergreen trees to 5 m high, they have glossy green leaves and star-shaped fragrant flowers.

Origin: East Asia, probably China.

Varieties: Imperial and Unshiu — popular in frosty areas, cropping early to late autumn; Emperor — large, easily peeled, delicious fruit in autumn, not for coastal areas; Ellendale — popular late autumn variety, more correctly known as a tangor (mandarin-orange hybrid); Seminole — a tangelo (tangerine-pomelo hybrid), very sweet and spectacular as a tub specimen.

Planting: Plant in full sun, in well-composted soil. Mandarins grow very easily in tubs and make excellent and highly decorative evergreen trees for small gardens and courtyards.

Cultivation: Keep your trees well-watered. Mulch and feed in spring and autumn with citrus food. Protect from fruit fly, to which mandarins are particularly susceptible.

Harvesting: Pick as required when ripe, for eating or cooking in marmalades, preserves, as crystallised fruits at Christmas time or in long, cool summer drinks.

Orange

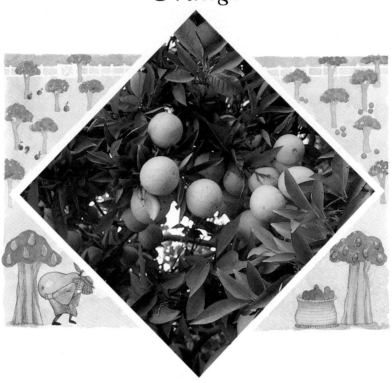

Also known as sweet orange, this much-loved, elegant, evergreen tree (*Citrus sinensis* and *C. aurantium*) has exquisitely scented flowers in spring. It does best in Mediterranean climates where it will reach 5–6 m.

Origin: China.

Varieties: Valencia — the most popular, with very juicy fruit from spring to autumn. Washington Navel — excellent quality, usually seedless fruit, late autumn to winter; blood oranges — sweet, juicy flesh.

Planting: Plant in full sun, in well-composted soil. Orange trees can be grown in frost-prone areas if you plant them in tubs and keep them in a greenhouse-like situation in winter, moving outside in warm weather.

Cultivation: Keep well-watered in hot weather. Mulch and feed in spring and autumn with citrus food. Protect from fruit fly and black spot.

Harvesting: Pick ripe fruit as required. For the highest vitamin C content, eat or drink juice within 10–15 minutes of cutting fruit open. Oranges also make the best marmalades, taste delicious as a liqueur, as crystallised fruit, in cakes, jellies and desserts, or cooked with poultry, roast meats or rice dishes.

SUMMER FRUITS
decorative and delicious

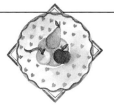

Summer fruits are as decorative as they are delicious. Most have spectacular and fragrant spring blossoms, while the bare branches of deciduous fruit trees in winter have a special beauty of their own.

Climate, Position and Soil

Deciduous fruit trees do well in cool temperate districts but should not be grown in late frost areas, as frosts in spring can injure or kill flowers and leaf buds. In coastal areas, where fruit fly is active, early maturing varieties should be considered. Consult your nurseryman or State department of agriculture representative as to the best types of fruit for your area.

All deciduous trees should be grown in a location with good air circulation and full sun. Good drainage is essential. They will grow on a variety of soils but organic matter such as compost is a valuable addition to poor sandy soil.

Planting

Plant deciduous trees in winter, when they are dormant. The trees may be bought bare-rooted or as potted plants.

The term bare-rooted means without soil on the roots. Make sure you don't allow the roots to dry out.

Dig a hole large enough to take the roots without crowding. Before planting, cut back broken or damaged roots. Spread roots out naturally, outwards and downwards. Plant trees just below the nursery soil mark, keeping the bud union well above soil level. Half fill the hole with crumbly topsoil and tread it firmly. Then fill the hole to ground level with more topsoil, treading it down firmly while doing so. Do not fertilise. Keep well-watered and spread a good mulch away from the stem to help conserve moisture.

Management

In soils of average fertility, nitrogen is likely to be the element most needed for deciduous trees. Apply a mixed fertiliser which contains about 10 per cent nitrogen annually in late winter or early spring. For young trees up to 5 years old, apply fertiliser at the rate of 500 g per tree for each year of the tree's age. A surface mulch of compost and rotted animal manure will also benefit the tree.

PRUNING TO A VASE SHAPE

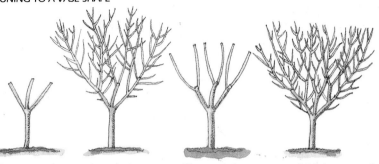

1) tree pruned to three main limbs after first year

2) second-year growth

3) pruned after second-year growth

4) third-year growth

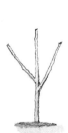

Newly-planted vase-shaped tree

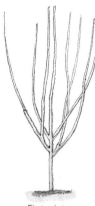

First winter before pruning

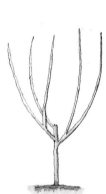

After pruning

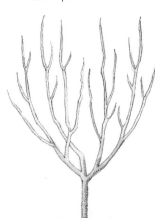

Second winter

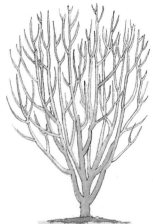

Mature vase-shape

After planting, cut back the young tree to about 40 cm high to encourage the development of three main limbs. A vase shape is best for most deciduous trees. Prune trees hard for the first few years to make a sturdy framework and to shape the tree.

Remove strong inward growing shoots annually at winter pruning. This allows more sunlight to reach the tree and encourages flowers and fruit. When pruning full-bearing trees it is important to remove all dead and diseased wood. Prune all deciduous fruit trees, except cherries, in winter. Cherries should be pruned in spring, just prior to leaf development.

Different kinds of fruit trees bear their fruits in different ways and it is important to know the bearing wood for each kind before pruning. Detailed pruning bulletins on individual fruit trees are available from your State department of agriculture.

THE BIG CHILL
Why some trees need cold weather

Deciduous fruit trees such as apples, pears, peaches, plums and cherries go dormant each year during autumn and winter. They do this in order to survive the months of freezing temperatures they're programmed to expect and without which they will not grow or fruit well. This need for low temperatures varies from species to species and is known as the *chilling requirement*. It is measured as the total number of hours below 10 degrees that the tree needs. Most stone and pome fruits have a high chilling requirement (about one thousand hours) and will not produce fruit of high quality where winters are mild. However, there are some varieties with lower chilling requirements and these should be sought out if you live in a mild climate.

Controlling Diseases and Pests

Apple and Pear Scab: Raised green or black areas appear on fruit. Burn infected fruit and leaves and spray with a fungicide.

Apple Powdery Mildew: Grey powdery substance appears on the underside of leaves. Spray with a recommended fungicide.

Brown Rot: This is a very destructive disease. Fruit shrinks and brown areas appear. Destroy affected fruit and spray with a fungicide.

There are several insect pests which the home gardener needs to watch out for.

Aphids: Tiny insects such as woolly aphids, cherry aphids, and green and black peach aphids may be a serious problem. When they appear, spray with insecticide and observe the withholding period.

Codling Moth: Small caterpillars feed near cores of fruit. Remove and destroy all infected fruit and spray trees with a recommended treatment throughout spring and summer. Control is mandatory by law.

Fruit Fly: See entry under Citrus Trees p. 8.

San José Scale: This can be a severe pest on deciduous trees. Scale covering the adult is greyish with a dark area in the centre. It feeds on the trunk, limbs, twigs and occasionally the fruit. Spray your tree thoroughly with an appropriate insecticide and observe the withholding period.

Apple

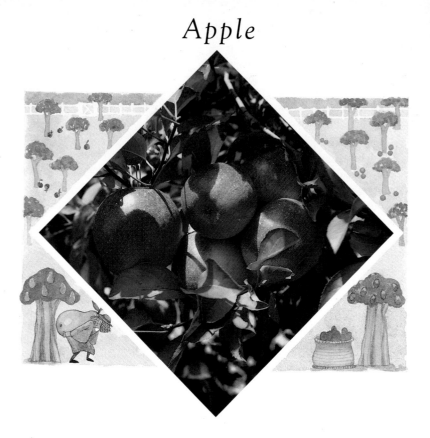

Apples (*Malus pumila*) are hardy deciduous trees growing to 5 m with beautiful blossom. Two varieties flowering concurrently are needed for pollination. Apples grow in temperate to cold climates.

Origin: Europe and Western Asia.

Varieties: Early fruiting — Willie Sharp, Earliblaze; mid-season — Spartan, Jonathan, Delicious and Golden Delicious; late — Granny Smith, a favourite both for eating fresh and cooking, with excellent keeping qualities.

Planting: Plant between mid-autumn and early spring, in full sun and loamy well-drained soil.

Cultivation: Water well even after harvest, so the following year's fruit sets well. Mulch with compost or poultry manure. Protect from codling moth and fruit fly.

Harvesting: Fruit takes 12–16 weeks to form. Thinning the crop in early summer can encourage fruiting every year rather than every alternate year, a problem with some varieties. Do not leave apples on the tree too long, as they lose their keeping qualities. Culinary uses are many — in jams, jellies, cakes, pies, wines (calvados is an apple brandy from France).

Apricot

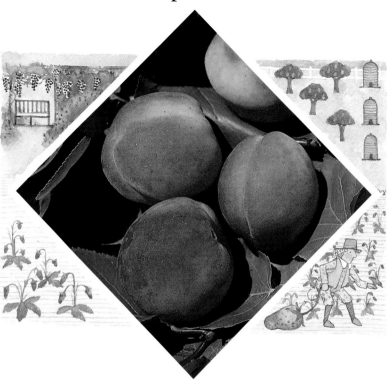

A pricots (*Prunus armeniaca*) are very adaptable as to climate but taste especially delicious when grown in areas with warm summers and cool winters. They are attractive deciduous trees to 5 m with exquisite, scented white blossom in spring.

Origin: China.

Varieties: Coastal areas — Glengarry and Caselin; cool highland and inland districts — Trevatt, Bulida and Moorpark.

Planting: Plant midwinter in full sun. They will grow in a wide range of soils. All varieties are self-fertile so it is not necessary to plant two trees for pollination.

Cultivation: Keep well-watered all year, especially from spring to autumn. Fertilise annually with citrus food and mulch with poultry manure in autumn. Thin fruit in spring and prune in early summer. Protect from attack by fruit fly.

Harvesting: Apricot trees crop 4–5 years after planting and should continue for up to 40 years. For the best flavour, pick mature, well-coloured fruit in midsummer. Apricots make excellent jams, preserves and drinks, as well as tasting delicious eaten fresh or dried.

Cherry

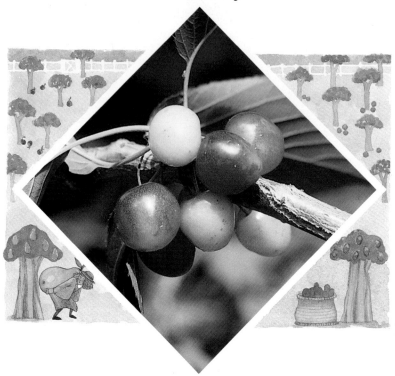

Cherry trees (*Prunus avium*) are among the most beautiful of all fruit trees. They thrive in cool areas with mild summers, growing 6 m high and wide.

Origin: Temperate areas in the northern hemisphere.

Varieties: Early — Burgsdorf and Early Lyons (dark red fruit) will cross-pollinate; mid-season — Rons Seedling (deep red fruit) will cross-pollinate with Early Lyons, Napolean and Florence (light-coloured fruit) will cross-pollinate; cold districts — Morello (a sour cherry, best for preserving) is self-fertile.

Planting: Plant in early winter, in deep, well-drained, loamy soil. Avoid heavy or wet soil and choose a position protected from wind. Most cherries are self-sterile, so plant two kinds.

Cultivation: Keep well-watered all year round; do not use a watering system such as a sprinkler which will dampen and damage fruit. Feed with a fertiliser high in nitrogen in mid-winter and dress with superphosphate in autumn. Prune only lightly in spring at bud-swell stage.

Harvesting: Trees crop when 3–4 years old. Pick cherries when fully ripe, about 6 weeks after flowering.

Fig

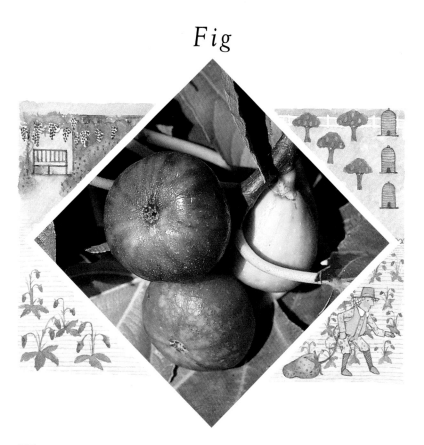

Figs (*Ficus carica*) have been cultivated for thousands of years. They
are very adaptable to climate range
but do best in subtropical and temperate inland areas. Mature trees tolerate frosts.

Origin: Asia.

Varieties: Black Genoa (purple skin
and red flesh); Brown Turkey (purple-
brown skin and flesh); White Adriatic
(green skin and pink flesh, excellent
for jam making).

Planting: Plant during winter when
trees, being deciduous, are dormant.
Plant in full sun in deep, moist soil.
Only one tree is needed.

Cultivation: Keep well-watered and
mulched. Feed with citrus food high
in nitrogen in early spring and midsummer. Prune lightly each year to
encourage growth of fruit-bearing laterals, so tree remains at 4–5 m high
for ease of harvesting. It is usually
necessary to grow figs under nets.

Harvesting: Trees bear fruit 4 years
after planting and produce two crops
a year, in early summer and again in
late summer or early autumn. Fruit
ripens over a long period, so check
tree daily and pick fruit when fully
mature and soft. Delicious fresh, dried
or made into jam.

Nectarine and Peach

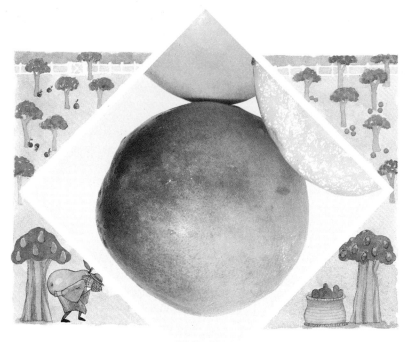

As their botanical names imply, nectarines (*Prunus persica* var. *nucipersica*) and peaches (*Prunus persica*) belong to the same species and their cultural requirements are identical. The main difference between them is their skin — nectarines are smooth-skinned while peaches have downy skins. Both are deciduous trees to 6 m with decorative pink blossom in spring. They do best in temperate climates with warm summers and cold winters. Most varieties are self-fertile so only one tree is needed. Many ornamental hybrids are cultivated only for their blossom, their fruit being useless, so be sure to check with your local nurseryman before buying anything. Peaches have been cultivated in China since around 2500 BC and have been celebrated in screens and paintings for centuries. They are extremely attractive in formal spring flower arrangements. New miniature hybrid forms make them particularly appropriate for courtyards and small inner city gardens.

Origin: China.

Varieties: Nectarines — Goldmine (delicious white flesh, mid-season crop, thrives in all districts); Sunred and Sunlite (yellow flesh, good early

Nectarine and Peach

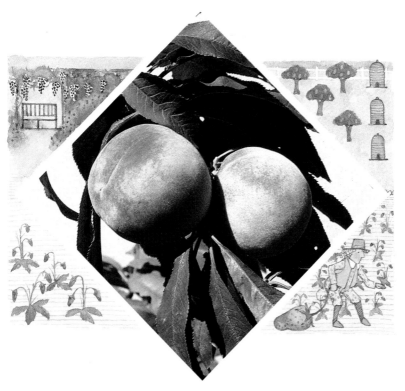

varieties for coastal districts). Peaches for coastal districts — White Shanghai; Flordasum (yellow clingstone), Maravilha (white-fleshed), Cardinal and Hiland (both yellow, medium-sized clingstones); peaches for cool highland areas — Redhaven (yellow semi-clingstone), Loring (firm, yellow freestone) and Fragar (delicious white clingstone). J. H. Hale, a yellow free-stone, needs cross-pollination by other varieties such as Blackburn and Malehaven.

Planting: Plant during early winter in full sun, in any well-drained soil — deep sandy loam is best.

Cultivation: Keep well-watered all year. Feed with mixed fertiliser in late winter and again in early summer. Mulch with compost or well-rotted manure. Prune in winter to a vase shape, retaining the shoots formed in the previous year. Protect from attack by aphids and fruit fly.

Harvesting: Trees start to bear 4 years after planting. Thin crop in early summer. Pick fruit when fully ripe and handle with care, as flesh bruises easily. Excellent eaten fresh, dried, in jams, preserves or purées. Nectarines are usually eaten with their skin; peaches are usually peeled before eating.

Pear

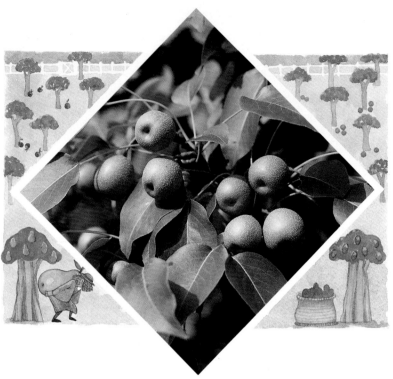

The pear (*Pyrus communis*) is one of the longest-lived, hardiest fruit trees. Large deciduous trees to 12 m, they need a mild summer and cool to cold winters.

Origin: Temperate areas of Europe.
Varieties: Williams — known as Bartlett when canned, the most popular variety for eating and cooking, with white, juicy flesh and yellow fruit from late January, will cross-pollinate with Beurre Bosc — long cinnamon-coloured pear, excellent quality, regular, heavy cropper with moderate keeping quality; Packham's Triumph mid-season, good quality, keeps very well, will cross-pollinate with Josephine — good quality but needs perfect growing conditions.

Planting: Plant midwinter in full sun, in deep, well-drained, slightly acid soil. Two varieties are needed for cross-pollination.
Cultivation: Keep well-watered. Feed with fertiliser high in nitrogen in late winter. Mulch with compost. Prune to a vase shape. Protect from fruit fly and codling moth.
Harvesting: Trees will bear 4–5 years after planting, for up to 50 years. Pick fruit while still firm so that final ripening occurs off the tree.

Persimmon

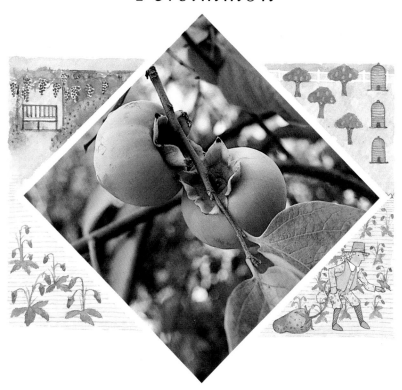

The ornamental persimmon (*Diospyros kaki*) is a deciduous tree growing 5–10 m, with a wide climate tolerance from subtropical to cool highland areas. Handsome, glossy leaves turn beautiful autumn colours, and fruit is a glowing orange.

Origin: Asia.

Varieties: Dai Dai Maru and Hachiya both produce good quality crops without cross-pollination.

Planting: Plant potted trees any time of year, bare-rooted trees in winter. Choose a sheltered position in full sun with deep, rich, well-drained soil. A highly decorative tree at all times of the year, a persimmon makes a good specimen planting.

Cultivation: Keep well-watered and feed with mixed fertiliser low in nitrogen in late winter and again in midsummer. Prune only lightly to an open vase shape. Protect from fruit fly.

Harvesting: Trees start cropping 3 years after planting. Pick fruit late summer or autumn when coloured but still firm and allow to soften indoors for a few days. Delicious fresh for breakfast or cooked in purées, jams, sauces and desserts. They also go well with roast poultry or meat, and can be frozen for storage.

Plum

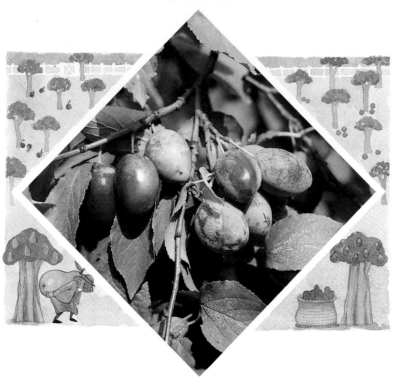

Plums are deciduous trees to 9 m which bear exquisite white blossom in spring. There are two main varieties — the European plum (*Prunus domestica*) and the Japanese plum (*P. salicina*).

Origin: North America to Japan.

Varieties: European plums — Angelina, President and Grand Duke, all cross-pollinate with each other. Japanese plums — Narrabeen (yellow flesh) and Maripo (blood-red flesh) will cross-pollinate; Santa Rosa (red-fleshed) is self-fertile.

Planting: Plant during winter in full sun in deep, loamy soil. Plums require cross-pollination of the same group — Japanese and European varieties are not compatible.

Cultivation: Keep well-watered but not waterlogged all year round. Feed with mixed fertiliser and mulch with compost or well-rotted manure. Little pruning is needed, as plum trees are mostly self-shaping.

Harvesting: Thin fruit in early summer and leave to mature on tree. Fruits are rich in minerals and Vitamin A (recommended as a protection against skin cancer by some skin specialists). Plums taste superb fresh or cooked in jams and tarts.

Quince

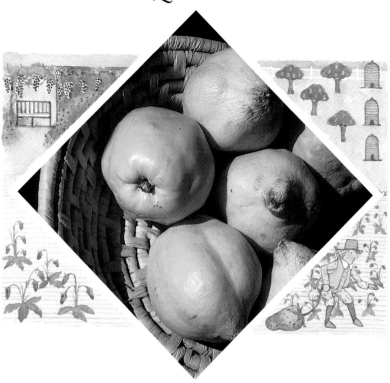

Very adaptable, hardy deciduous trees to 4 m, quinces (*Cydonia oblonga*) grow from the subtropics to cool, highland areas. Attractive spring flowers are followed by yellow fruits in late summer or autumn depending on the cultivar.

Origin: Eastern Europe and Asia.

Varieties: Champion, De Vranja, Pineapple and Smyrna — fruit tastes better when cross-pollinated with another variety but a single tree can crop well.

Planting: Plant during winter in a sheltered position in full sun, in deep, rich soil with plenty of moisture.

Cultivation: Keep well-watered and mulched. Feed with mixed fertiliser in late winter and mid-summer. Protect from fruit fly and codling moth. Prune to a vase shape and pinch out tips of lateral branches. Fruit appears on new season's growth so be careful not to prune this.

Harvesting: Trees crop 5 years after planting, in summer. Fruit is popular for bottling and jam-making; squares of quince jelly, set with almonds, taste delicious as an after-dinner sweet. Quinces are also used to make jams, preserves, tarts and potent home-made liqueurs.

TROPICAL FRUITS
for the gourmet gardener

Like most fruit trees, tropical fruits are often ornamental as well as being useful and many make attractive large specimen shrubs or trees. They are ideal for gardeners who enjoy eating fresh fruit salad or making their own jams and preserves with slightly more unusual ingredients — guava jam, for example, is excellent, while breadfruit purée makes a delicious dessert with ice-cream.

Climate, Position and Soil
Tropical fruits thrive in tropical temperatures but many can be grown in temperate zones which are frost-free. Some will even tolerate light frosts once they are mature trees, if they are planted in full sun in a position sheltered from winds. Wind not only damages branches and fruit, it also dries out the soil and tropical fruits need plenty of water all year round. Some tropical trees have a spreading habit so make sure you plant where they will have plenty of room — see individual entries for details.

Planting
Make the planting hole wide and shallow rather than deep and narrow.

Place compost or plant food in the base of the hole, cover with a layer of soil if using plant food (so that roots don't come in direct contact with chemicals which may burn them) and stake plant if your area is subject to sudden tropical storms. Water in well and mulch, to conserve water, keep weeds down and provide a soft landing bed for those fruits that fall off the tree when ripe.

Management
Tropical trees require ample water. If planting in tropical zones, the wet season may well take care of this for part of the year but trees may require extra feeding if nutrients are being leached out of the soil. Feed with citrus food and choose compost or leaf-mould as your mulch if possible.

Controlling Diseases and Pests
Diseases and pests thrive in tropical conditions with high temperatures, humidity and lots of leafy growth to feed off. There are preventive measures you can take, particularly where diseases are concerned. Burn any leaves that look infected; place healthy twigs and clippings on top of

your ordinary mulch around the base of fruit trees — this keeps mulch in place during downpours and assists drainage in the soil especially during the wet season. Dispersing water efficiently helps stop water-borne viruses and spores from splashing against tree trunks and lessens the likelihood of root rot. Growing trees under netting is probably the only way to protect them from vermin such as flying foxes, rats and crows.

Anthracnose: Small raised brown spots appear on fruit near harvest time. Spray with a recommended treatment and prune tree to an open shape to prevent recurrence.

Brown Spot: Large brown spots appear on fruit and leaves, and leaves may fall. Spray tree with a recommended fungicide.

Collar Rot: See entry under Citrus Trees p. 8.

Powdery Mildew: A white powdery substance appears on leaves. Spray with a fungicide.

Root Rots: Very prevalent in tropical zones. Plants become weak and wilt. Treat with a soil drench. Can be avoided with good drainage.

There are several insect pests you will need to protect your tropical fruit from, in addition to the vermin mentioned above.

Fruit Fly: This is often the most serious pest attacking tropical fruit. See entry under Citrus Trees p. 8.

Fruit Spotting Bug: This causes blemishes in fruit skin, especially avo-

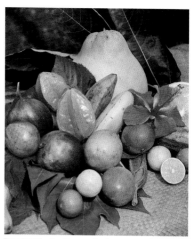
Tropical fruits, the perfect summer dessert

cados. Spray with a recommended insecticide when you first notice bugs.

Leaf-eating Caterpillars: If irregular chunks have been chewed out of your leaves, caterpillars may need to be removed, by hand if possible; otherwise, spray with insecticide.

Mealy Bugs: See entry under Citrus Trees p. 8.

Monolepta Beetle: Yellow and red beetles swarm over trees. Spray with an appropriate insecticide.

NOTE: In some States, there are particular legal requirements for growing bananas. In New South Wales, for example, in coastal regions north of the Hunter River, gardeners need a permit to plant or move a banana tree. Check with your State department of agriculture to find out what is required by law in your district.

Avocado

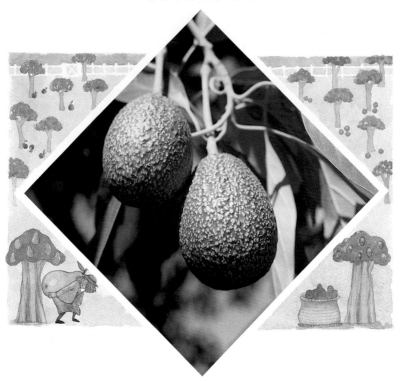

A vocados (*Persea americana*) are small to medium-sized evergreen trees that do best in non-coastal areas where there is a warm to hot summer followed by a mild frost-free winter.

Origin: Central America.

Varieties: Hass, Sharwil and Fuerte are all self-fertile but planting pollinator varieties does ensure maximum cropping — Hass and Sharwil are compatible cross-pollinators; Wurtz is a smaller variety which is cross-pollinated by Sharwil.

Planting: During late summer or late winter plant commercially grafted trees (seedlings are unreliable crop-pers) in a sunny, sheltered position with deep, well-composted soil.

Cultivation: Keep well-watered. Mulch regularly and avoid cultivation near the trunk as roots are close to soil surface. Feed several times in spring and summer with fertiliser rich in nitrogen. Prune to an upright or spreading shape, 5–10 m high.

Harvesting: Grafted trees produce after 3 years. Avocados do not ripen well on the tree, so harvest when fruit is fully formed and ripen for a few days indoors inside a brown paper bag with a lemon. Serve halved, with lemon juice and black pepper.

Banana

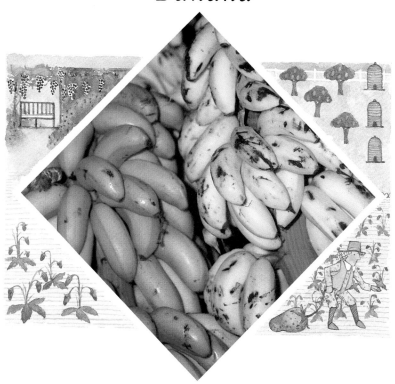

The banana plant (*Musa* species) is a very large herb growing 3–6 m. It thrives in tropical areas but will tolerate colder conditions if protected from wind and frost.

Origin: South-east Asia.

Varieties: Cavendish, Williams (good for cooler areas), Grand Michel, Lady Finger and Sugar.

Planting: Plant any time in tropical areas or in early summer in cooler districts. Choose a position in full sun, with lots of space and rich, well-drained soil.

Cultivation: Keep well-watered in summer. Feed with a complete fertil-iser three times a year once new growth appears. As the parent plant grows, suckers will grow out from the roots. Leave only one or two to replace the parent plant after fruiting.

Harvesting: Tree should crop about 1 year after planting. About a month after each 'hand' appears, it can be protected with a plastic cover slipped over and loosely tied at the top, leaving the bottom open. Cut bananas when still green, about 3–6 months after they first appear, depending on variety. After the harvest, cut down the parent plant leaving one or two suckers to grow to maturity.

31

Breadfruit

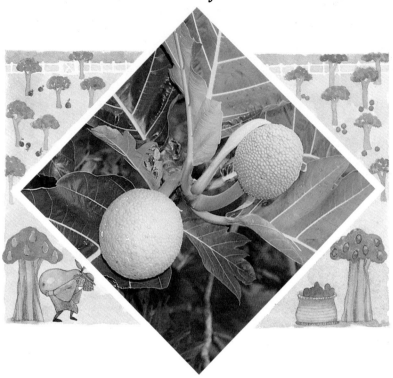

readfruit (*Artocarpus incisus* syn. *A. altilis*) looks like a large melon with sweet yellow flesh. The tree grows to 15 m with distinctive dark green leaves. It will grow only in tropical zones. Breadfruit first became famous with the mutiny on the *Bounty*. Sir Joseph Banks, the famous botanist, was interested in growing exotic plants as additional food sources. Accordingly, Captain Bligh was sent out to take breadfruit from Tahiti to the West Indies, to provide cheap food for the plantation slaves. Prevented by the mutiny, he succeeded four years later, on the *Providence*. Several spec-

imens also reached Kew Gardens.

Origin: China and Malaysia.

Varieties: No named cultivars seem to be available as yet.

Planting: Plant cuttings or shoots in an open position with full sun and rich, moist soil. An ideal courtyard plant with very decorative foliage similar to a *Monstera deliciosa*.

Cultivation: Keep well-watered at all times.

Harvesting: Fruit ripens in the summer wet season. Cook as for potatoes (bake, fry or boil and mash) or mash raw fruit to use in desserts. Seeds may also be cooked and eaten.

Custard Apple

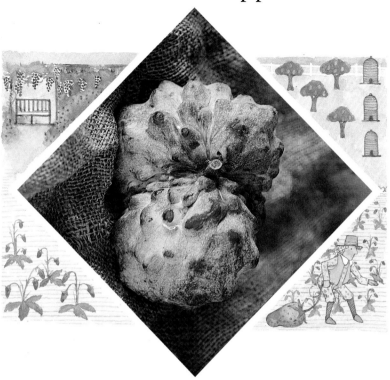

The custard apple (*Annona cherimola*) is a subtropical fruit also known as the sugar apple. It grows 6 m high with a spreading habit in a warm humid climate but is adaptable to temperate zones.

Origin: South America.

Varieties: African Pride — the most popular; Pink's Mammoth.

Planting: Plant grafted nursery trees in spring and summer, in well-drained soil. Choose a position with plenty of space. Some varieties need another plant for cross-pollination, so check with your local nursery.

Cultivation: Keep well-watered at all times. Feed with citrus food four times a year. Prune trees to a vase shape and protect from fruit fly and frost damage. Prune carefully as fruit appears on each season's new growth. Remove any branches that touch the ground.

Harvesting: Trees bear fruit 3–6 years after planting, depending on variety. Fruit ripens over a long period in spring and summer and tastes delicious eaten fresh in fruit salads, as fruit pulp served with cream or ice-cream, as the basis for ice-creams and sherbets, as a refreshing, cool drink or in cakes and desserts.

Guava

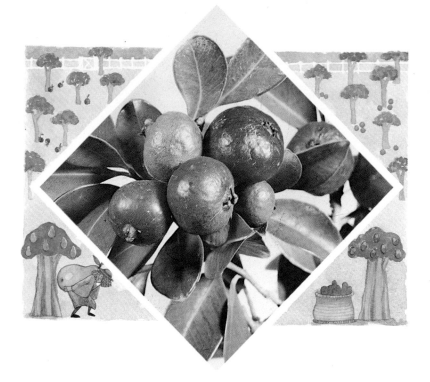

The commmon guava (*Psidium guajava*) thrives in tropical climates where it can reach 5–9 m. It is, however, adaptable to temperate conditions. The tree bears large white flowers and yellow oval fruit with a fine flavour.

Origin: Haiti.

Varieties: There are no named cultivars available as yet. Another species is available, *P. cattleianum*, the cherry guava, which is better for cold climates and makes a good tub specimen. It is the preferred form grown in New Zealand.

Planting: Plant cuttings any time of year in any soil in a sunny position sheltered from wind.

Cultivation: Keep well-watered in hot weather. Feed with citrus food in midwinter. Protect from fruit fly. Guavas are usually problem-free. Prune after fruiting — trees are usually self-shaping but branches may need shortening for ease of harvest.

Harvesting: About 18 months after planting, fruit should appear. Pick in autumn when fully ripe — delicious eaten fresh, made into an excellent jelly, used in fruit compotes and salads. Guavas are believed to contain more vitamin C than oranges.

Jackfruit

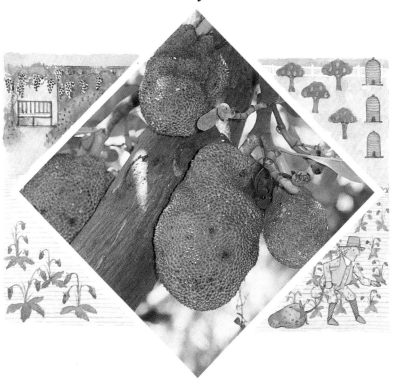

Jackfruit or jakfruit (*Artocarpus heterophyllus* syn. *A. integrifolia*) is the same genus as breadfruit with similar cultivation needs. It is a handsome evergreen tree growing to 20 m with catkin-like flowers and attractive, deeply-lobed leaves.

Origin: Malaysia and India.

Varieties: There are no named cultivars available as yet, but there are soft-skinned and firm-skinned types in Asian markets.

Planting: Plant in deep, rich, well-drained soil. The plant thrives in very humid conditions.

Cultivation: Keep your trees well-watered, especially during hot weather, otherwise these are low-maintenance trees.

Harvesting: Fruit takes 6–8 months to ripen. It is said to be the largest fruit in the world, and may reach 1 m long and up to 20 kg in weight. You can eat the sweet pulp raw, cooked or dried, after first removing the rind. Mashed pulp may be added to curries and other hot, spicy dishes, fried in oil as a side dish or added to cool drinks. Seeds can be roasted. This fruit tends to be an acquired taste, as not everyone immediately appreciates its pungent quality.

Lychee

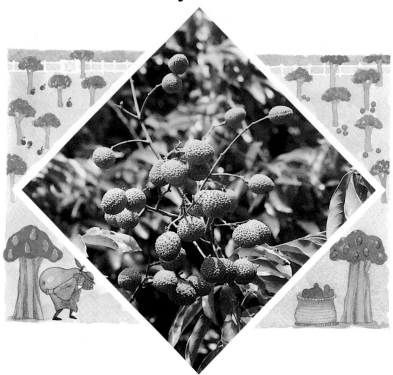

The lychee (*Litchi chinensis*) is an attractive, slow-growing tree to 12 m high, with decorative leaves and bunches of oval fruit. Fruit has mottled red skin enclosing a delicious white flesh. Lychees thrive in high humidity and hot summers.

Origin: China.

Varieties: Tai So — bright red fruit; Heak Ip — smooth-skinned, dull red fruit; No Mai Chi — yellow fruit; Wai Chi — highly recommended fruit.

Planting: Plant young grafted trees from a nursery in a position sheltered from wind with full sun and deep, well-drained compost-rich soil.

Cultivation: Water well in summer and mulch to conserve moisture and keep down weeds. Feed annually with blood and bone. Protect from leaf burn with shadecloth during the hottest months. Little pruning is required as lychees are usually self-shaping. Remove tangled inner branches if it becomes necessary.

Harvesting: Trees will crop 4–6 years after planting. In summer, pick fruit in clusters every few days when richly coloured. They taste delicious added to fruit salad or served with ice-cream. A favourite Chinese dessert fruit in restaurants.

Mango

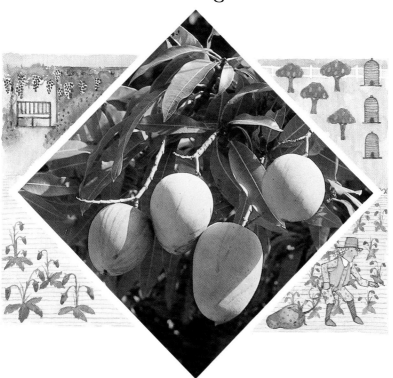

The mango tree (*Mangifera indica*) is an attractive evergreen reaching 6–12 m high and 8 m wide. It needs a tropical climate with a dry period during spring flowering for fruit to set properly.

Origin: Indonesia and Malaysia.

Varieties: Kensington — pinkish-orange fruit of excellent quality; Common (syn. Turpentine) — yellow-green fruit, good yield.

Planting: Plant during the spring months. Choose a position with full sun and rich, well-drained soil. Protect from wind.

Cultivation: Keep very well-watered until established. Feed with mixed fertiliser four times a year. Prune immediately after fruiting, thinning out branches to the strongest.

Harvesting: Trees start bearing 4–6 years after planting. Pick fruit in clusters when richly coloured, from late spring to autumn. Test for ripeness by choosing one fruit and cutting it open — flesh should be firm, juicy and a rich yellow colour (though some varieties are red, pale yellow or orange). An excellent source of vitamins A, B and C, mangoes are usually eaten fresh (good for breakfast) and added to fruit salads and punches.

Passionfruit

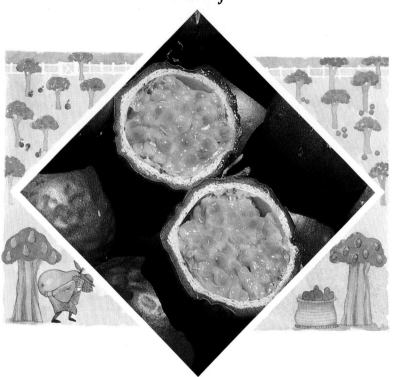

Perennial vines, passionfruit (*Passiflora* species) are often grown as much for their flowers as their fruit. They have a wide climatic tolerance, depending on variety.

Origin: South America.

Varieties: Purple (*P. edulis*) — the most widely cultivated in Australia, has several named cultivars, e.g. Redlands Triangular, Redlands Pink and Lacey, will grow in tropical and temperate regions; golden passionfruit (*P. edulis flavicarpa*) — a stronger vine but more susceptible to cold, best in the tropics and subtropics; banana passionfruit (*P. mollissima*) — yellow fruit, suitable only for tropical areas; granadilla (*P. quadrangularis*) — very large fruit, suitable for tropical and subtropical areas.

Planting: Plant in spring and summer in any well-drained soil, with full sun and support, preferably a fence or trellis running north to south.

Cultivation: Keep well-watered. Pinch tips of new growth to encourage laterals. Prune each spring. Feed monthly with fertiliser high in nitrogen and mulch annually with manure.

Harvesting: Vines should crop 6–8 months after planting. Pick fruit when ripe — wrinkled and fully coloured.

Pawpaw

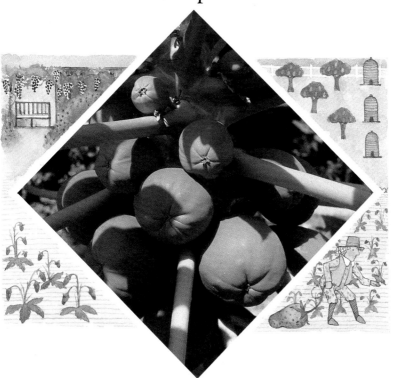

Also known as papaw, papaya and papita, pawpaws (*Carica papaya*) thrive in tropical areas but can grow in temperate, frost-free regions. They are fast-growing, attractive, evergreen trees to 7 m.

Origin: South America.

Varieties: Fijian (small red), Red Thailand (long and slim) and Babaco.

Planting: Plant in full sun in well-drained, deep, composted soil in a position sheltered from wind — against a wall or fence is ideal. A male and female tree are needed for pollination. Hybrid bisexual trees can be bought from nurseries if you prefer to plant only one tree.

Cultivation: Keep well-watered and mulch to conserve moisture. Pawpaws are heavy feeders and need plenty of fertiliser three times a year. Protect from powdery mildew and dieback.

Harvesting: Trees start cropping 15–18 months after planting and continue for 5 years. Pick fruit when fully coloured during the summer months. When picking, be careful to avoid a milky substance that oozes from the fruit stalks — it contains an enzyme that causes skin irritation in some people. Pawpaws contain vitamins A and C.

Pineapple

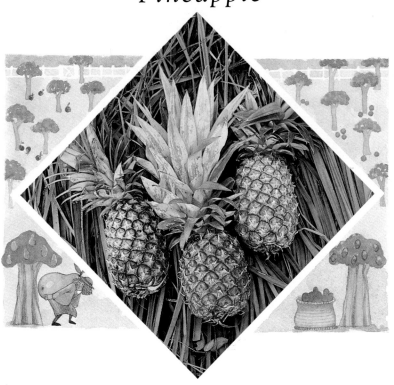

Pineapples (*Ananas comosus*) are herbacious perennials, growing 60–120 cm high only in tropical and frost-free subtropical zones; in cooler areas, grow in a greenhouse.

Origin: South America.

Varieties: Smooth-leaf Cayenne — very juicy fruit; Common Queen and Ripley Queen — more compact plants with sweeter, less juicy fruit.

Planting: Plant during spring, in a sheltered well-drained position in full sun. They prefer sandy, well-composted loam and acidic soil. Pineapples can be attractive houseplants. Use a clay pot and give plenty of water. Use a fine misting spray to water leaves daily. Do not place at eye level, as leaves are long and spiky.

Cultivation: Mulch with compost and grass clippings. Feed monthly during summer with fertiliser high in nitrogen, watering in well. Prune in late winter. Protect garden from nematodes by removing and burning any infected plants.

Harvesting: Plants should crop 2 years after planting. Pick fruit when ripe and well-coloured, in summer. Pineapple contains an enzyme which helps us to digest protein, so it goes well with meat such as ham.

Rosella

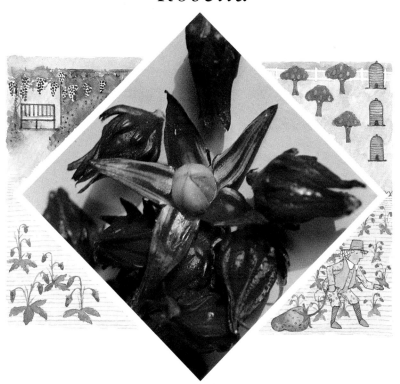

Rosellas (*Hibiscus sabdariffa*) are grown in tropical and subtropical regions. An annual growing 1.5–2 m with yellow flowers, rosellas have red or yellow fruit.

Origin: Hawaii and the West Indies.

Varieties: There are no named varieties available as yet.

Planting: Sow seeds in punnets in spring and keep damp. Plant seedlings in full sun in well-drained, composted soil in a position protected from wind. A long summer is needed for plants to fruit well, so while rosellas tolerate a wide range of soil types, their climatic requirements are quite specific

and they are only suitable for tropical and subtropical areas.

Cultivation: Feed with fertiliser high in nitrogen. Keep well-watered but not waterlogged. Stake to protect from wind damage in districts where this is likely.

Harvesting: Rosellas should be ready for picking 10–12 weeks after transplanting. Pick fruit when fully ripe and well-coloured and use the juicy pulp around the seeds for stewing, to make delicious jams and jellies somewhat similar to cranberry sauce in flavour. Pulp can also be added to refreshing summer drinks.

Tamarillo

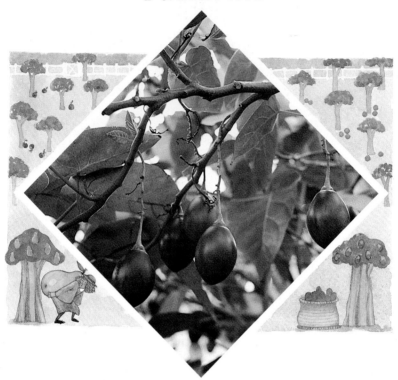

The tamarillo or tree tomato (*Cyphomandra betacea*) is an evergreen growing 2–4 m tall, with thick stems and large leaves. It grows quite easily in tropical and frost-free temperate climates.

Origin: South America.

Varieties: There seem to be no named cultivars but red and more rarely, yellow kinds are available.

Planting: Plant winter seed or summer cuttings in a sunny, sheltered position with good drainage.

Cultivation: Shorten seedling plants to about 1 m high to encourage branching. Keep well-watered in summer and mulch with compost or manure. Feed with fertiliser once in winter and again in summer. Prune late winter to remove damaged or diseased branches. Roots are shallow so do not weed close by.

Harvesting: Fruiting starts about 18 months after planting and continues from autumn to the following spring. Fruit can be refrigerated for several weeks. It tastes similar to a conventional tomato and can be used in similar ways — fresh in salads, entrées and soups, or cooked in casseroles, side dishes, jams, preserves and highly spiced, delicious fruit chutneys.

BERRIES
and other fruits

I n this chapter, berries and other fruits that don't fit neatly into a particular category, are discussed.

Climate, Position and Soil

Berry fruits — blackcurrants and redcurrants, blueberries, boysenberries, cranberries, loganberries and raspberries — all require full sun, good drainage and cold winters to crop well.

As these plants all have shallow roots close to the soil surface, mulching is particularly important, to keep weeds down without damaging the plant, retain soil moisture in dry seasons and, if mulching with compost, provide a year-round supply of organic plant food.

Other fruits require different climates: olives, grapes and pomegranates thrive in a warmer Mediterranean climate, with long hot summers and cool winters; kiwi fruit and melons grow in temperate zones; while strawberries and mulberries are very adaptable and grow in a wide climatic range.

For planting and management, see individual entries following.

Controlling Diseases and Pests

Berry fruits are usually fairly hardy and, given the right conditions, will thrive without too many problems. They are, however, attractive to birds and may need protection with netting.

Anthracnose: See entry under Tropical Fruits p. 29.

Grey Mould: Fruit rots and is covered with a grey mouldy substance. Remove diseased fruits.

Leaf Spot: Brown irregular-shaped patches appear on leaves. Remove diseased leaves.

Aphids: See entry under Summer Fruits p. 17.

Fruit Fly: See entry under Citrus Trees p. 8.

Light Brown Apple Moth: The caterpillar attacks grapes. Spray with a recommended insecticide.

Mulberry Leaf Spot: Spray with a recommended fungicide.

Blackcurrant

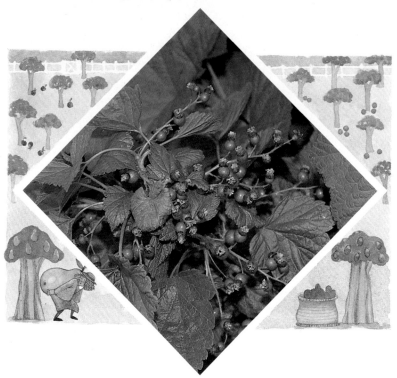

Blackcurrants (*Ribes nigra*) are a deciduous bush fruit rather than a trailing berry growing to 2 m. They are ideal for cool to cold climates and need cold winters to fruit well.

Origin: Europe, Britain and parts of northern Asia.

Varieties: Goliath, Baldwin, Carter's Black Champion, Dunnet's, Black Naples.

Planting: Plant cuttings in winter in full sun. Choose a position sheltered from wind with moist, well-drained, compost-rich and acidic soil. Improve poor soil by adding fertiliser.

Cultivation: Keep well-watered. Remove weeds before planting if possible, otherwise avoid weeding too deeply and damaging roots near the soil surface. Add complete fertiliser in winter and mulch with compost or well-rotted animal manure. Prune to a vase shape, retaining the previous two years' canes which will produce fruit. Remove older canes by cutting at the plant base. Protect from aphids.

Harvesting: Blackcurrants crop in early summer. Pick when fully ripe if eating fresh. If cooking, choose fruit that is slightly under-ripe. This fruit tastes delicious made into jam. Pick when fruit is black.

Blueberry

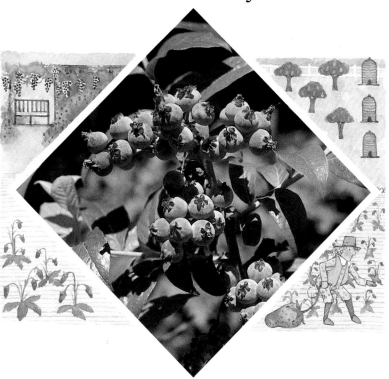

The blueberry (*Vaccinium* species) is a deciduous bush with ornamental spring flowers which thrives in temperate climates with a cold winter.

Origin: North America and Asia.

Varieties: There are several forms: Highbush (*V. corymbosum*) — most common in Australia, grows to 4 m and has large fruit; Rabbiteye (*V. ashei*) — to 6 m; and Lowbush (*V. Augustifolium*) — to 45 cm. Cultivars: Burlington — the most popular; Dixi — not for wet areas; Stanley — good dessert fruit.

Planting: Plant cuttings during spring in sun or semi-shade, in an open position with moist, very acid soil (pH 4.5).

Cultivation: Keep well-watered after flowering, while fruit is developing. Protect from birds with netting. Feed in late winter or early spring with complete balanced fertiliser such as azalea food. Plants are shallow-rooted so avoid weeding deeply. When plants are about 4 years old, prune in winter, leaving previous year's growth which will produce fruit.

Harvesting: Plants crop 3–6 years after planting, in late spring to early summer. Pick when fruit is slightly under-ripe.

Boysenberry

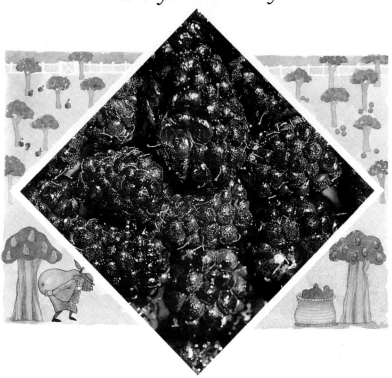

Boysenberries (*Rubus* species) are a hybrid developed from the trailing blackberry. Dark red berries grow on a vigorous deciduous shrub to 3 m. Adaptable as to climate, they need a cool winter to crop well.

Origin: Uncertain, possibly United States of America.

Varieties: There are no named varieties available as yet.

Planting: Plant rooted tip cuttings during late winter in any compost-rich, well-drained soil. Choose a sheltered position against a fence or trellis in sun or semi-shade.

Cultivation: Keep well-watered during spring. Feed annually with citrus food in late winter or early spring and mulch with compost or well-rotted animal manure. Weeds and grasses should be removed from the soil before planting, otherwise weed carefully so as not to disturb the surface roots.

Harvesting: Shrubs crop 2 years after planting in early to late summer. Pick ripe fruit when a deep colour and use in drinks, jams, preserves or fresh in summer desserts. Summer puddings are particularly delicious when made with a combination of summer fruits, such as boysenberries, blackberries, loganberries, blueberries, raspberries.

Cranberry

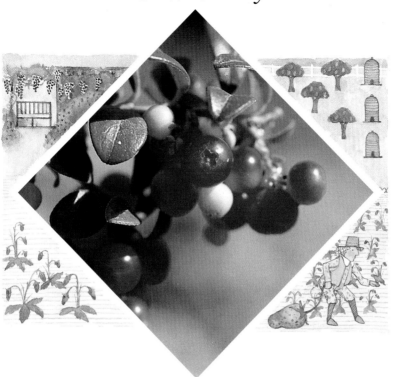

R elated to the blueberry, cranberries (*Vaccinium macrocarpum*) are
compact, evergreen shrubs with dainty
white or pink blossom and scarlet fruit.
They thrive in cold wet areas.

Origin: North America and Asia.

Varieties: There are no named cultivars available in Australia but several
have been developed in the USA
where cranberries are an important
commercial crop. Various forms of the
plant exist: the small cranberry (*V.
microcarpum*), the cowberry (*V. vitis-
idaea*), foxberry, partridgeberry and
ligonberry, available from specialist
nurseries only.

Planting: Plant cuttings at the end
of summer in damp, boggy, acidic soil
and water in very thoroughly.

Cultivation: Plants appreciate so
much water it is better for the gardener
to keep them flooded rather than
moist in spring, summer and autumn.
In winter, keep soil moist.

Harvesting: Cranberries bounce
when ripe, hence their other common
name, bounceberries. They store well
so are a valuable source of vitamin C.
These acid fruit can be used in many
ways — in jams, preserves, and the
well-known sauce. They also make
good pies and cakes.

Elderberry

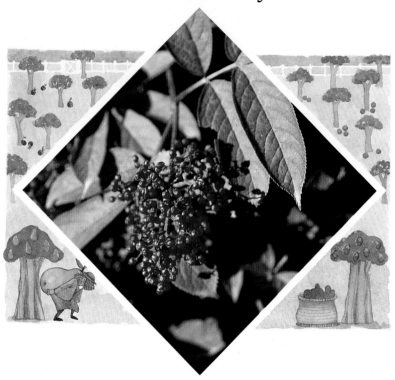

There are several forms of the elderberry (*Sambucus* species). Deciduous trees with bright green leaves and small, fragrant, white or pink flowers, they are adaptable to a wide range of climates.

Origin: Temperate and tropical areas of the world.

Varieties: American or Golden elderberry (*S. canadensis*) — two cultivars Monster and Ratty Red are being developed in Australia, growing to 4 m with very juicy fruit; European elderberry (*S. nigra*) — grows to 10 m, many cultivars available with variegated leaves that colour well in autumn; Western elderberry (*S. caerulea*) — to 3 m, very hardy, makes an excellent windbreak.

Planting: Plant cuttings during spring in any moist soil high in nitrogen, in sun or semi-shade.

Cultivation: Elderberries need very little attention. Prune in autumn to desired shape.

Harvesting: Berries turn black when ripe and should be picked in bunches rather than individually. Traditionally used in wine, champagne, preserves and jam, elderberries also taste delicious in pancakes, fritters and cooked fruit desserts.

Feijoa

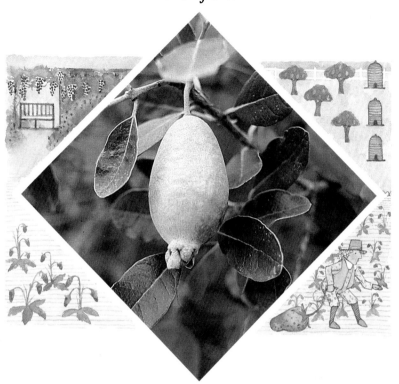

The feijoa (*Feijoa sellowiana*) is a very hardy evergreen tree growing 3–5 m, with ornamental red flowers and oval fruit. They grow well in subtropical zones but are adaptable to different climates.

Origin: South America.

Varieties: Coolidge, Mammoth and Triumph.

Planting: Plant seeds or cuttings in spring in moist, rich soil. Some kinds are self-fertilising but if planting from seed, plant two kinds to ensure pollination. Protect from frosts.

Cultivation: Keep well-watered and mulched. Avoid surface weeding near shallow roots which damage easily. Feed with citrus food in spring and summer. Prune older plants only if cropping lessens (feijoa are usually self-shaping). Protect from attack by fruit fly, scale, caterpillars and sooty mould.

Harvesting: Trees bear when 3 years old. In autumn fruit falls when ripe, so mulch around the tree with straw to protect fruit from bruising. Eat raw or as juice, or make into jams, preserves or chutneys. An excellent source of vitamin C, feijoas taste very like guavas and may be used in the same ways.

Gooseberry

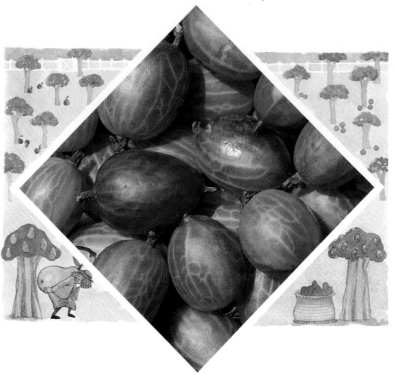

Gooseberries (*Ribes grossularia*) can grow in several forms, as upright bushes or more trailing plants. They have sharp thorns and are a deciduous shrub, thriving especially in areas which have cold winters.

Origin: North America.

Varieties: Roaring Lion — dark red; Crown Bob — red; Selection — yellow; Yorkshire Champion — yellow-green; Farmer's Glory — dark red.

Planting: Plant cuttings during winter in full sun, in a sheltered position with moist, compost-rich, well-drained, acidic soil. In city gardens, they can be trained against a wall, to save space.

Cultivation: Keep well-watered and weeded. Add complete fertiliser in winter and mulch with compost or well-rotted manure. Prune to an upright shape, unless training against a wall, in which case prune carefully to espalier the tree. Protect from frosts, anthracnose and powdery mildew.

Harvesting: Gooseberries ripen in early summer. In France they are used to make a superb sauce to go with mackerel; they can also be puréed and made into tarts and pies. Young leaves can taste delicious added to summer salads, as an alternative to lettuce.

Grapes

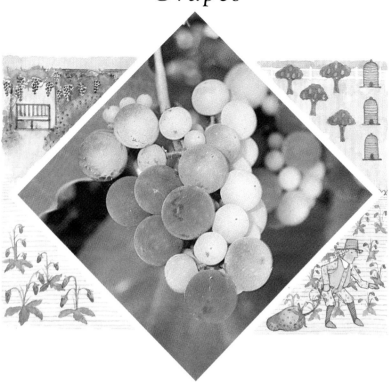

Cultivated for centuries, grapes (*Vitis vinifera*) grow on a deciduous vine that can reach 25 m high with support. Vines are very ornamental and modern cultivars have a wide climatic tolerance.

Origin: Caucasian areas, western Asia, southern Europe, Africa.

Varieties: White — Sultana (vigorous vine, sweet, seedless fruit), Golden Muscat (coastal regions); black — Cardinal (dry inland areas, large fruit), Red Emperor (vigorous vine, large fruit which stores well), Concord (cool climates).

Planting: Plant during winter in full sun, in fertile, well-drained soil with compost added before planting.

Cultivation: Grapes need very little feeding. Pruning is essential, depending on the shape you want — espaliered against a wall, trained to a fan shape or up a trellis or grown without support as a bush. Fruit crops on one-year-old wood which grows out of two-year-old wood, so gardeners need to prune carefully.

Harvesting: Vines crop 2–3 years after planting. Different varieties can be enjoyed for different purposes — eaten fresh or dried as raisins, or used for winemaking or juice.

Kiwi Fruit

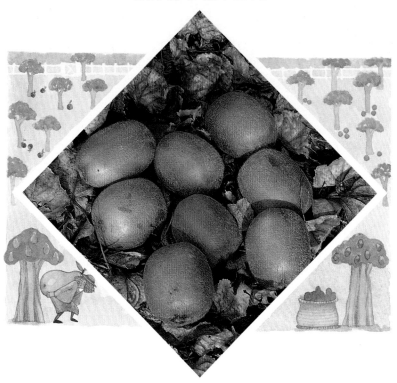

Also known as Chinese gooseberries, kiwi fruit (*Actinidia chinensis*) is a large deciduous vine thriving in temperate climates. It is very high in vitamin C, surpassing even citrus fruits.

Origin: China.

Varieties: Hasward — most popular; Bruno — heavier crops earlier in the season.

Planting: Plant both male and female plants in winter next to a support such as a trellis or pergola. Plant in full sun, in deep, well-drained, composted loam, sheltered from wind.

Cultivation: Keep well-watered and feed annually in winter with citrus food. Protect vines from frost or hot winds. Fruit grows at tips of each year's new growth so prune in winter after your crop has finished or you will cut off next year's harvest. Protect from fruit fly.

Harvesting: Vines crop 4–5 years after planting, in late autumn or early winter. Pick when it is soft as a ripe pear, or harvest when under-ripe and leave at room temperature until soft. Fruit tastes delicious fresh or frozen, in jams, pickles, chutneys, or desserts and salads. It is also very popular as a decoration for desserts.

Loganberry

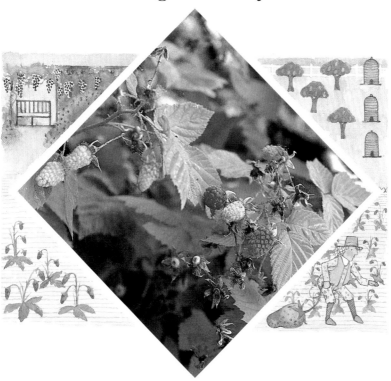

Thought to be a hybrid of the blackberry and the raspberry, *Rubus x loganobaccus* produces long arching canes, white blossom and delicious red fruit in temperate to cold climates with a cold winter.

Origin: United States of America.

Varieties: There are no named cultivars available in Australia as yet.

Planting: Plant rooted cuttings in winter when dormant, in a position with full sun, against a trellis or fence sheltered from winds with well-drained, very rich soil.

Cultivation: Mulch with compost or well-rotted animal manure. Feed with citrus food in late winter or early spring. Prune after fruiting which occurs on the previous year's growth. Weeds and grasses should be removed before planting, otherwise weed carefully to avoid damaging fragile roots close to the soil surface.

Harvesting: Canes crop 2 years after planting in summer and early autumn. Use as for blackberries and raspberries, in jams, sauces and preserves; desserts such as summer puddings, home-made ice-creams and sherbets; jellies, hot fruit desserts; as a filling for pancakes, pikelets, cakes, scones, pies and tarts.

Melon

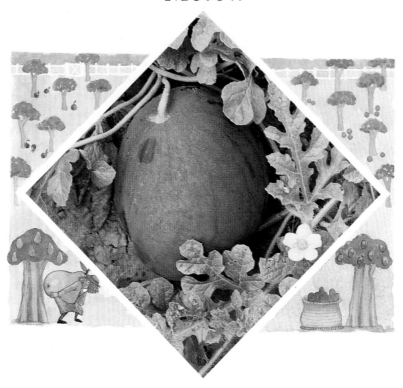

Melons belong to the cucurbit family which includes cucumbers, gourds and pumpkins. They thrive in temperate to tropical areas.

Origin: Asia or tropical Africa.

Varieties: Rockmelons, also known as cantaloupes (*Cucumis melo cantaloupensis*) — Hales Best (the most popular, disease resistant); Dixie Jumbo (excellent flavour); Supersprint (round fruit, heavy cropping); Honey Dew (oval fruit with sweet green flesh); watermelons (*Citrullus lanatus* syn. *C. vulgaris*) — Candy Red Hawkesbury (large fruit, hardy vines); Sugar Baby (small round fruit); Sunnyboy (attractively striped rind, excellent flavoured flesh).

Planting: Sow seeds direct or in punnets in spring or summer in well-composted soil. Choose a position with plenty of room to spread out or train vines against a trellis.

Cultivation: Keep well-watered. Feed with soluble plant food monthly after flowering starts.

Harvesting: Vines should crop 14–16 weeks after planting. Leave melons to ripen fully on the vine. Rockmelons should come away from the stalk easily while watermelons develop a slightly bumpy rind when ripe.

Mulberry

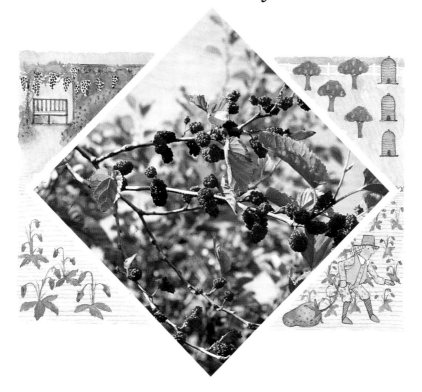

Mulberries (*Morus* species) are deciduous trees from Iran growing 6–10 m. They have a wide climatic tolerance. Their beautiful leaves make them attractive shade trees for suburban gardens.

Origin: Iran, the Caucasus or possibly Nepal — authorities differ.

Varieties: Black English (M. *nigra*) — best for cooler areas; Hicks Fancy (M. *rubra*) — a white variety for warmer areas.

Planting: Plant autumn cuttings during winter in full sun, in deep, well-drained loam. Mulberries can grow in containers but in the open garden need plenty of room to spread. Make sure you avoid planting anywhere near a washing line, as berries (and birds) can ruin your laundry.

Cultivation: Keep well-watered in dry seasons. Protect from birds. There are no special pruning requirements — fruit will appear on new growth each year.

Harvesting: Trees crop 2–3 years after planting. Pick fruit in summer when fully ripe and eat fairly soon after, as mulberries do not store particularly well. Mulberries are excellent eaten fresh or made into jams, jellies and pies.

Olive

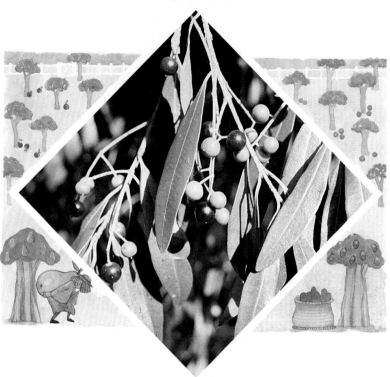

The ornamental olive tree (*Olea europea*) has been cultivated for centuries in Mediterranean countries for its oil, used for lamp light, cooking and religious ceremonies. It is a small evergreen tree growing 2–12 m depending on how you prune it.

Origin: Asia Minor and Greece, according to some authorities, Egypt according to others.

Varieties: There are over 700 cultivars grown for different purposes, green pickling, ripe pickling or for oil production — Mission (fruit and oil), Manzanillo, Verdale and Sevillano are some available in Australia.

Planting: Plant during autumn or spring in full sun, in well-drained, fertile, crumbly soil.

Cultivation: Olives are very shallow-rooted so keep well-watered and mulched at all times. Feed annually with citrus food in late winter. Prune to a comfortable height for harvesting. Protect from black scale and frost.

Harvesting: Trees crop 5 years after planting. Fruit bruises easily so handle with care. For green pickling, harvest when fruit is pale green or yellow; for ripe pickling, pick black olives when fully coloured and store in jars between layers of salt for 2 months.

Pomegranate

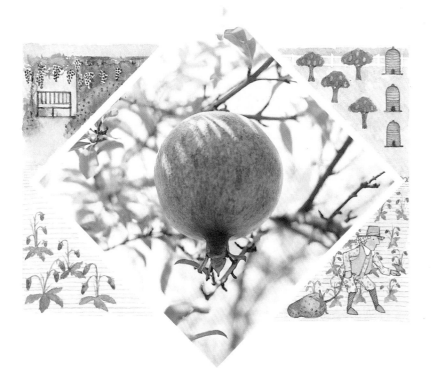

Loved by the ancient Greeks, the pomegranate (*Punica granatum*) is an attractive deciduous tree to 7 m with glossy leaves and orange-red spring flowers. They need long, hot summers without rain or humidity, and mild winters.

Origin: Mediterranean area, as far east as India.

Varieties: There are no named cultivars available in Australia at the moment, though large and dwarf forms can be found.

Planting: Plant cuttings or suckers in winter, in deep, well-drained soil. Dwarf varieties make good tub speci-

mens, while the larger kinds can be planted as a useful hedge.

Cultivation: Keep well-watered in spring. Feed annually in winter with citrus food. Remove suckers from around base of tree and prune crowded branches to let in air and light. Protect from fruit fly and frost.

Harvesting: Trees crop 5–6 years after planting. Pick fruit in late autumn to early winter when slightly under-ripe and allow to ripen fully indoors in a cool, well-ventilated area. Fruit looks magnificent in bowls — as the skin varies from yellow to purple and seems to glow.

Raspberry

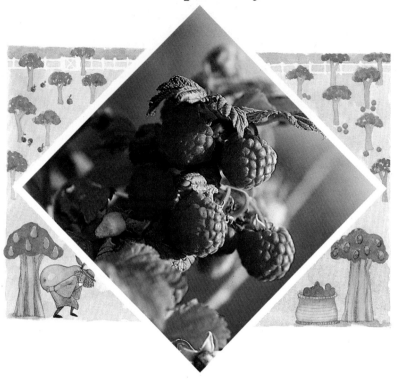

Raspberries (*Rubus idaeus*) are hardy, deciduous shrubs suited for cool climates with mild summers and cold winters. They make marvellous summer dessert fruits — white, red or black according to variety. New hybrids are being developed.

Origin: Europe, Scandinavia, Great Britain, north and east Asia.

Varieties: Willamette, Heritage, Everbearer, Exton Late.

Planting: Plant suckers in winter in a position with full sun and shelter from winds. Support with a trellis. Soil should be well-drained, moist and slightly acid.

Cultivation: Keep weeds and grasses down with a mulch of compost and well-rotted animal manure. Feed with citrus food in late winter or early spring and prune after fruiting — fruit grows on one-year-old canes, so be careful to remove only the old canes.

Harvesting: Canes crop 2 years after planting, in summer and autumn. Fruit is superb served fresh with cream or ice-cream; made into jams, preserves and jellies; served with other fruits such as pears and peaches; whipped into creamy, puréed desserts set in a mould; or simply sandwiched between the layers of a sponge cake.

Redcurrant

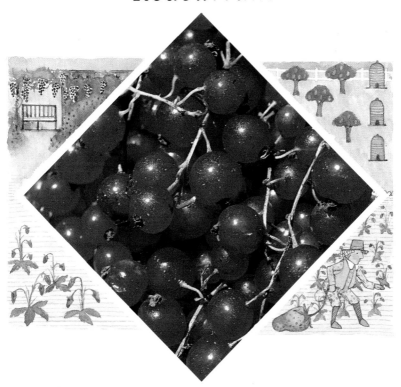

Redcurrants (*Ribes rubrum*) are very similar to blackcurrants — a cold climate, deciduous trailing berry, ideal for mountainous or table-land areas.

Origin: Europe, east Asia, Manchuria and also Siberia.

Varieties: Fays Prolific, Red Dutch, La Versailles.

Planting: Plant cuttings during winter in full sun in a sheltered position with moist, compost-rich, well-drained, acidic soil. Choose a position where bushes will be protected from frost, which damages flowers and affects fruit quality.

Cultivation: Keep well-watered and weeded. Add complete fertiliser in winter and mulch with compost or well-rotted animal manure. Prune in winter and again in summer retaining the previous year's canes which will produce the fruit. Shrubs can be trained into a variety of shapes, depending on planting position — against walls and fences, along wires, as vase- or fan-shaped bushes.

Harvesting: Canes bear in late spring and early summer. Pick berries when fully ripe if eating fresh and slightly under-ripe if using for cooking or preserving.

Strawberry

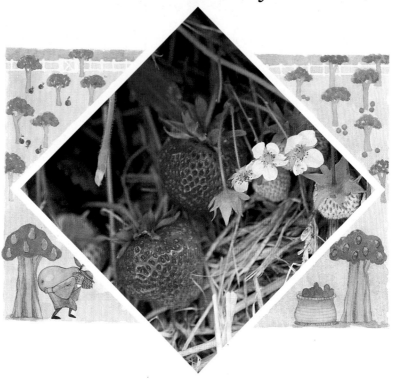

Easy to grow, strawberries (*Fragaria* species) are very rewarding, producing a good crop in their first year. They adapt to different climates.

Origin: Europe, northern Asia, north America.

Varieties: Contact your State agriculture department for certified virus-free varieties recommended for your particular area.

Planting: Plant during autumn or winter in raised beds or containers, spacing plants 30 cm apart. Strawberries need well-drained, composted soil and full sun.

Cultivation: Mulch with compost or grass clippings to suppress weeds and keep soil temperature constant. Alternatively, cover with black horticultural polythene in which slits are cut for the plants to grow through. Feed with soluble plant food every 2–3 weeks. Keep well-watered until berries start to colour, then gradually decrease watering.

Harvesting: Plants crop 6 months after planting in spring and summer. Pick berries when fully ripe. Berries which have matured in full sun have been found to contain higher levels of vitamin C than those grown in semi-shade.

USEFUL EXTRAS
general gardening information

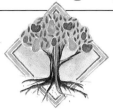

There's more to successful gardening than choosing the right plants for your area. Every gardener should be aware of the type of soil in the garden and how to improve it and keep it free from weeds.

Compost

Every garden needs a source of rich, organically nourishing compost. Why? All plants need carbon, hydrogen and oxygen, which they get from water and the air. They also need large amounts of calcium, magnesium, nitrogen, phosphorus, potassium and sulphur; and small amounts of trace elements — boron, cobalt, chlorine, copper, iron, manganese, molybdenum, sodium and zinc. A balance of these is essential for plants to thrive, especially introduced species designed for other climates and soils.

Gardeners can vastly improve garden soil and so plant performance, by adding manures and chemical or organic fertilisers like peatmoss, sawdust or leaf-mould. They can also use compost, which is a lot cheaper and helps solve local garbage disposal problems by recycling waste products. These days there are a number of commercial compost tumblers on the market but an old-fashioned compost heap at the back of the garden is cheap and easy.

A three-sided enclosure of concrete building blocks makes the perfect spot in an out-of-the-way corner disguised by low shrubs. Position it so that the back faces the house.

You don't need a concrete base — compost ripens much faster in contact with bare earth where worms can get to it. Use any organic material that will rot (leaves, grass clippings, kitchen scraps). Add a sprinkling of soil and perhaps some blood and bone between layers. Keep everything damp, turn with a fork occasionally and speed the process by covering your pile with a polythene sheet until it has 'ripened' through. In summer material should be ready for use after about two months. When weather is colder, the process will take four or five months. Ensure that plant material put in the compost heap is free from disease.

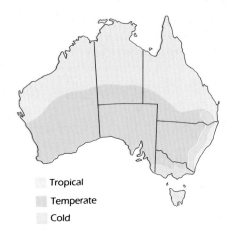

Tropical
Temperate
Cold

Australia's Climatic Zones

The vast majority of Australians are city dwellers living in temperate coastal areas. Most of the instructions in this book, on what to do around the garden, are aimed at these. However, we have included extra information that relates more specifically to tropical or cold areas. If in doubt about your type of climatic zone, see map, or consult your nursery.

Mulching

Why spend half your gardening time weeding and watering when it isn't necessary at all? If you put down a loose layer of organic material over the soil surface this will: reduce soil temperature in hot weather by as much as 15°C; reduce evaporation of moisture; smother weed seedlings; and last but not least, provide plant food as it slowly breaks down. Some are plain, some are fancy and some are even free, depending on where you live. The

best mulch for fruit trees is compost. Select from leaves, grass clippings, well-rotted animal manure, seaweed or straw.

These are organic mulches which were once a living thing or part of it. They rot down over time, slowly releasing valuable plant foods as they do, encouraging worms and other useful soil organisms and gradually improving the texture of the soil. Organic mulches should be replaced periodically — that is replaced, not just topped up, so that roots are forced to grow upward to feed. This replacement is usually done every year in spring and at the same time you need to add a nitrogen-rich fertiliser to the soil to compensate for the nitrogen that soil bacteria use in decomposing the mulch itself.

How do mulches work?

Water conservation: Mulches conserve soil water in two ways. Firstly, they reduce evaporation by shading the surface of the soil from hot direct sunlight thus keeping the ground considerably cooler. Secondly, they prevent winds from drying out the surface. You'll need to water much less often — a saving of time and money, not to mention our precious and limited water resources. Your plants will enjoy the cooler, moister conditions around their roots as well.

When you do water, organic mulches absorb and hold water for later use by plants. The uneven surface of most mulches prevents rapid run-off, improving the infiltration of the rainwater into the soil where it is needed. Obviously, materials such as plastic sheeting (used to grow strawberries) do not have this advantage.

Weed suppression: A mulch will completely smother emerging weed seedlings and without sunlight they will wither and die. Seeds that germinate beneath the mulch at a later stage will suffer the same fate. If you use grass clippings, manure or compost as a mulch, you must be sure they do not contain weed seeds or these will germinate and grow as usual.

Slow-release feeding: Organic mulches also provide plant food as they rot and some are considerably richer than others, compost being the best. Some organic mulches rot down quickly while others are fairly slow. Quick rotting mulches include: compost, grass clippings, manure, leaves and seaweed. Slower rotting mulches are nut shells and kernels and wood or bark chip. The slower a mulch breaks down, the less nutritious and useful it will be.

Where can you find an excellent source of mulch? Garden centres, landscape material suppliers or your own garden, which can supply grass clippings, twigs, sticks, leaves and prunings of all sorts which should never be thrown out. Rather, you should stash them under the shrubbery where they will break down in time, just as they do in the bush.

Chipping or mulch-making machines can be ordered through larger garden centres and hardware stores and come in a wide range of sizes and prices. Standing usually on a tripod base, they are much like an old-fashioned mincing machine. You feed the garden litter into a chute and finely chopped mulch pours out the other end into a wheelbarrow.

Mulch can be applied all year round, though the best time is late spring after the soil has warmed up a little. The soil should be thoroughly and deeply soaked before mulching and loose mulches should be applied 4–5 cm thick. Mulches much deeper than this yield little additional benefit. Keep all mulches at least 10 cm away from plant stems or you will lose many through the fungus collar rot.

Mulches should be replaced each year, for natural decomposition and the activities of earthworms soon incorporate them into the soil.

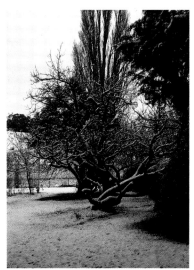

Fruit trees can be grown across a wide climatic range.

63

Index